Acknowledgments

I have found that in life there are lessons in places you don't expect and teachers you don't know you'll learn from. The some of the most powerful experiences in life are when you're just living it. You go about your day to day and the seemingly mundane can be where the key to purpose may be. I have been blessed with amazing teachers; from an active family of 5 unique, creative and awe-inspiring siblings (Shekinah, Zoe, Zachary and Samuel) and two driven and committed parents. I've taken so much in and continue to be taught by them constantly. Even in the small things. I bathe in the wisdom gained from new friends and connections, I soak in new revelation for days. We become a reflection of our teachers and the wisdom we seek.

I see the world around me seeking for purpose and hoping for direction and I know that I am to do what I can with all I have to assist however I can. This book continues a journey as I use my experiences and what I've learned to prayerfully inspire and encourage you! I'm glad to bring you along. There's destiny ahead; even though it will be a challenge it can be reached, come with me and we'll Face To The Future.

Face To The Future

Caleb Vaughn

Cover design by Glave Photography LLC

Forward and Edited by Michael and Sheila Vaughn

The Journey

Back To The Table

Center Of Wonder

One Plus One Is One

I'm Not A Mama's Boy I'm A Blessed Son

Everyone Else Is Taken

Exceed And Defeat The Expectations

Best Effort No Matter The Audience

Set Your Time By Me

Fuel Up

Face To The Future

<u>Forward</u>

Author, student, athlete, prolific communicator, intrapreneur, loyal friend, son, man of God! This is the person that we know as Caleb Vaughn. Caleb has always been someone that is very introspective. He goes in deep and comes out with ideas, insights and information that is a blessing to those that he interacts with. He has a memory better than an elephant and therefore is able to make each person that he meets feel special. He remembers the details of when he met them, what they enjoy and something about who they are. He loves music and reacting to it. This is an extension of who he is, fun loving and enjoying life. You are in for a special experience as you read this book. There are nuggets from this book that will give you things to think about that could change your life if you let it. Enjoy this experience and get ready to gather some insights from this wonderful young man that also happens to be our son!

- Micheal Vaughn (Dad)

What a treasure to call him my son. Caleb Michael Vaughn my first born, purpose-filled, impactful man of God. When I first laid eyes on him my heart filled with such love, joy and wonder. God had given me the amazing assignment to mother this beautiful person. Little did I know that Caleb would not only mark our lives but he would grow and make positive impact everywhere he found himself. From grade school to grad school he is still pursuing life with integrity and excellence. I couldn't be more pleased of the man my son has become.

-   Sheila Vaughn (Mom)

<u>Back To The Table</u>

It's never too late to start living and until you're gone you always have an opportunity to engage your purpose. There are people whose lives depend on your fulfillment and activation of your purpose, as ultimately your purpose is NOT for you.

March 11, 2019; the day I turned 27. I didn't know anything about 27. I guess it's the beginning of my "late" 20s. Seven (7) years before when I turned 20; this decade seemed so…mysterious…so exciting. Throughout my teenage years it was something to look forward to. Now I'm looking at my last three (3) years of this decade and pushing towards a future of full excitement, joy and purpose. I notice a lot of twenty somethings live like all the purpose in life ends at 30. I was never overtly conscious of this mindset, but I did live like it sometimes. There's an idea that many experiences and opportunities must be had before 30 or you're doing life wrong. There's an idea that by the time your 30 you must have obtained at least a bachelor's degree, gotten married had a kid a or two, bought a house and hitting an upward trajectory in your job field. All of this by 30. Then the idea sets in that because your twenties can be filled with so much of the freedom of mobility that many want in their teens that being a 20 something will be the highlight and pinnacle of your existence. I'm still in my twenties and am looking to maximize every day and opportunity I have with my life, people and my experiences. At times I do get caught up thinking about "deadlines" but I'm not nervous about what 30 will bring. The beauty in looking to maximize where you are is that when you get to places that you want to go, you'll be able to draw on the previous knowledge and experience gained. You're output will be greater though because of what you've gone through.

As well there's also no reason to live on the time table of other people. It's easy to get wrapped up in how other people are accomplishing different things and seeing different shifts in their lives that you may want for your own. You may ask "when is my turn" or "what am I doing wrong." Those questions often can lead to more frustration and discontentment. The evil in the mindset that one can be entrapped in through this line of thought is that by considering and focusing on what you aren't getting or why you aren't there. Ironically you can make yourself more unavailable for the shift you seek in your life because you're more focused on why you aren't there rather than preparing yourself to get there. Preparation is the biggest difference between people who want greatness and great things for their lives, as opposed to people who live in greatness and walk out great lives. Even if you are "late" or you're in the middle of the bliss that so many other people express to want you still must responsibly handle where you are intentionally.

Center Of Wonder

I'm from Rochester NY and I lived in Buffalo NY for 7 years with 4 ½ in college and a few years of postgrad working life. At one point in my sophomore year, a graduating senior who was a friend of mine told me about some of the great experiences that he was looking to do post grad as he accepted a job in Atlanta. Hearing all the amazing things to be expected in Atlanta began a wonder of getting to see and experience it. I also got to visit Toronto that year and it confirmed to me with so much world out there I would certainly have to move. I couldn't be confined to just life in one region when so much more of who I believe I am and what I was looking to experience or even just excited to explore would be outside of where I've always been. So much of maximizing who you are will come from what you learn outside of your comfort zone. I wasn't thinking that I was going to move for purpose, but I knew I was looking to grow and expand. Sometimes in life you have goals and desires but the only way to get to experience them is to go out and do them. A lot of people want to make life changes for themselves; whether it's deciding to be with a particular person for the rest of their life, going back to school, getting a new career or moving to a new city for a change of experiences and scenery. I did 3 of 4 in the same month in 2018. I moved 1100 miles, began a new job and started graduate school. It's been a journey in adjusting and being malleable for expectations as I've created a new set of norms and routines for my life. Many people would like to make similar changes in life, and here I'd like to offer ideas and advice of how to get there or go after similar goals.

To make a big move you must consider your motives for moving. If you're moving because it's a trendy place to be or because of a temporary situation where you're currently living isn't going your way moving might not be what you should do. Where a lot of people make mistakes for a big move is that they'll seek to move because "there's no good people" in their current city. Or "there's nothing to do". The issue with this mindset can be that these people forget themselves as the common denominator and when they do get to a new city it can be even MORE frustrating because they figured that they would enjoy the new place but end up in the SAME type of situation they thought they left.

When I was considering my move there were a few things that were specific about Atlanta that I wanted that Western NY wasn't going to provide. My desire for Atlanta began with a discussion with a graduating senior when I was a sophomore who was moving to Atlanta for a job opportunity. He told me about all the new experiences he was heading to and all the future opportunities he could expect to enjoy. Having grown up in Western NY the type of people and opportunities I was hearing that were in Atlanta were unlike what I had seen for myself. I desire to be a business executive who can mentor, create space for growth and I want to be able to directly bring in young bright business professionals specifically ones of color. Atlanta is a great place to be such an executive. It's not to say that Buffalo wouldn't afford the same type of role I'd look to exercise but as I'm looking to grow towards that the opportunities aren't as prevalent as in Atlanta.

My secondary reason for wanting to live in Atlanta is the weather. I completely dislike being cold and for a person who's grown up in Western NY and was born in the middle of a major snow storm I knew I didn't want to experience snow and subzero temperatures if I didn't have to. Even though the cold and snow are parts of winter that I've grown to "get used to" the weather was something I always wasn't a fan of. There was a serious threat of some sort of snow 8 months out of the year. I have experienced snow storms in April and September. In comparison to Western NY the Atlanta weather is a great mix of mild and hot. Being landlocked and a way from any major bodies of water humidity isn't factor like it is in Miami or Houston which are on the ocean. In my first winter I haven't experienced any snow at all. There might have been days that snow has come but I wasn't in that part of Atlanta and that snow didn't stick. The coldest days of my first winter was in the twenties. During my winters in Western NY the average temperature during the prime part of the winter would be in the mid to high twenties. Sometimes there were entire weeks where the temperature was even in the teens or lower. I would make a joke that "If the temperature was lower than my age, I'm too old to be outside." I also would say "If we can see your breath, we shouldn't see your skin." Now being that I live in Atlanta I've experienced 50s and 60s even as much as 70 in the middle of January and I'm enjoying it. Also, to note, it may be minor, but I've noticed that there are no rusty vehicles here the weather is wonderful for cars. In Western NY; salt used to help remove ice from roads also can corrode the metal on cars and can speed up the aging process of a vehicle. With my car here I've only washed it once in 7 months, I just KNOW that I've added years to the life of my car by moving. The weather is one of the major highlights of being in Atlanta and I struggle to appreciate it enough.

As I mentioned I transitioned into a new job and began graduate school as well. It's a lot to do just one of those things even aside from being in a new city. Getting ready for these transitions were not easy ones to make but daily I would investigate the programs in Atlanta I had applied to and stay on top of my deadlines. I would also reach out to the professors that would be teaching in the programs so that I could ensure that I was going to do everything I could to give myself the best chance to successfully move into further study. Fortunately, my acceptance and enrollment into my program came 5 months before I moved so I was able to have that part of my transition "checked off."

Having gotten into my program with a set date for the start of classes I was able to then focus on getting a new job in a new city. I wanted to move into a new role but stay in the same company. The organization that I had been part of offered stability and growth opportunity of which has helped foster what I'd like to implement as an executive. The very seeds of what I wanted my professional legacy were sewn in this organization. The challenge for me was that in my desire to move the position I was in at the time didn't exist in Atlanta. So, I had to investigate applying within the company to a new role and even department. That organization seeks to hire from within, but they can't place people where there is no room. I was very aggressive and stayed on the company's job board to see when a role would open. My primary goal in staying with the same organization was that I wouldn't have to also add transitioning into a new company in the list of transitions. This time period was great timing for me to enter a new role in the company as I had spent 2 years in my role to that point and had a strong handle of my functions.

Ultimately getting to make the transition to graduate school and a new role has meant that I had a lot of different things that I had to juggle with many tasks to complete as well as dates to be aware of. In order to be successful in doing all that I need I took a lot of notes of what I was looking to do. Even more than a checklist I would look create mini plans for how each of the tasks would get complete. I had a running list of the people I wanted to speak with regarding the new role. Another list of apartments and the places I wanted to get in contact with as well as making sure that I was focused in on the things that were still needing to be done where I was currently. Keeping a big picture in mind I made sure to make sure that I was still protecting myself if things didn't work out. This part of my transition was the part that gave me the most grief. I had everything set but I didn't have a job in Atlanta yet. I didn't think it would be wise to move and figure things out when I already had a stable situation in Buffalo and just move with whatever other timing that would end up coming. I had a couple of back up plans and alternatives if things didn't turn out as I had hoped.

I believe that as a single man, being able to take the chance and make a big move to a new city is wonderful opportunity to change scenery. The best thing about making a major move when you're single and no one depends on you is that there's even fewer moving parts in making the move, there's no one else to convince to also move and you don't also have to plan the logistics of others making the move with you as well. I think that single people sometimes get locked in their singleness and don't continue to pursue their goals and work in their purpose.

I believe that in a season where you're free to your own life you should do what you can to position yourself to go after the dreams. Sometimes life happens and we must delay our desires for our lives because other responsibilities take a precedent before some of the ones for your own life can be attended to. One day I look to be married and to be a father; knowing that I have certain career and educational aspirations as well as geographical desires the taking care of what I can first would allow me to enjoy what I hope to up front rather than having to hold back from the pursuit of those goals when I'd have the opportunity to. I decided not to be stuck and not live in delay.

To make a big move you must be intentional in planning. Plan, plan, plan. I created lists and laid out all the things that needed to be done and, in the time, that it needed to be done for me to make a successful move. I had several lists that were going but I knew the time frame that I wanted to move and knew that I was undertaking a lot in order to make that this move. A lot of people say that they want to change their life situation or experience different aspirations but do nothing to prepare to do so. A lot of people just "assume" that by hoping and wishing and even speaking that there will be the change they hope for, but they haven't done anything to move forward. It's great to aspire but you must have to do work to see the realization of your goals and dreams.

I've seen many people talk about the things that they wanted to do in life and never set their feet in motion. I like to be a person who goes for their goals with all that they have and won't allow themselves to be denied. I'm working on not being so frustrated when things don't work out, but I still push hard. When you want to make changes in your life get to finding out what it will take to move on to those changes being reality. Search for the resources, the people and that information that will lead you then execute. If you don't initially find an answer it's usually just that you haven't found the key. It's amazing what changes and how you can move forward once the key is found. Remember to plan, plan, plan and then execute!

One Plus One Is One

My parents have a daily routine in communication that just is amazing to me. Before my Dad goes to work, my parents talk together and pray, then sometime in the middle of the day my Dad will call my mom and they'll talk a little. To continue; my Dad will THEN call my mom on his way home and they'll chat. It doesn't stop there! When he gets home and checks in on all the people home (they have 5 kids and a dog) my parents then chat some more! I'm of the belief they have more discussion in bed before they got to sleep. But in all that communication they know each other incredibly well. There are no alarming surprises and lingering arguments. They can work through issues by being open and constantly checking in. I believe a lot of anger and issues in disagreements come from both miscommunication and not communicating at all. By being intentional in communication my parents keep those issues to a minimum. They often talk about being the best friend of the other and I believe that wholeheartedly. When you're engaging with someone you genuinely like to be around more than any other person, you'll do what you can to remain around them and engage harmoniously. It's an element that I hope to have in my own marriage.

I love to communicate, and I love to be part of encouraging others. I like to be part of helping them grow I get excited when I'm able to be the person that has the words to say that will help someone through where they are or being able to recognize them in their successes. I love to cheer on others and praise them. So, what better opportunity and experience would it be than to be able to daily do that with my wife?! One of the biggest things I look forward to in marriage is being able to do cute things for my wife and tell her all the wonderful things about herself. I look forward to the beautiful challenge it will be to come up with creative ideas and word placements in my speech to communicate an ever growing and maturing woman. A woman that I'd be blessed to forever be married to. I look forward to having to work out disagreements with a woman who has the same aim as I do but we're just trying to bring each other in to the other's perspective.

I've watched my parents do exactly that. My Dad pursued a relationship with my mother for two years because he just knew she was the one for him. He believed that God had revealed it to him that she would be his wife and went right on to basically make it known that that would be how things would go. Unfortunately, my mother did not hear from God the same way at the time and found my dad corny thus she was NOT interested. However, she made the mistake of allowing him to continue to talk to her and be her friend.

Eventually after he chilled out and no longer tried to make it happen it quickly turned around. I believe that part of why they are so intentional toward each other is because my Dad had to be so patient. Imagine being promised something and you are so incredibly sure that it will happen, but you must wait two years for it? How would you proceed in preparing for it? What would your perspective on that thing not coming into agreement with what you believe has been promised? I think a lot of people would've become bitter. Others would've given up even. I wonder how my father felt in that time to be honest I've never asked him. I must believe that it was incredibly frustrating but one thing that I know is that when it takes someone a long time to get something, or a lot of effort must be expended to get somewhere you appreciate what you were working towards a lot more. I believe that trying two-year season gave my father an appreciation for my mother that shows his commitment to her and why he refuses to do anything that would damage their marriage. I believe that those two year also showed my mom that she can be confident in her husband to the point she can bring all of herself to him. That time, that period. The space before they would be able to stand before the world and begin a walk to be remembered as they would create together fond memories that were the planting and watering of striking legacy. All would essentially be an investment that they wouldn't want to see a positive return from. They built a solid a strong foundation, they dug deep and firm roots and from what they have planted they continue to water. When one is vested in a project or any endeavor the more time and energy placed in and on that investment to see it be prosperous gives a greater appreciation for it. That is one of the many but most solid things I've seen when I watch my parents.

I don't have the typical type of relationship with my parents that many people have experienced. I have an excellent relationship with both my mom and my dad. I really can't think of anything, any struggle any doubt, any celebration that I didn't feel comfortable bringing to either one or both of them. They have been married for more than half of their lives and continue to do things that will keep them married the rest of their lives. I often marvel at how intentional they are in their efforts towards each other. They are constantly thinking about each other, and just looking to be a blessing to the other one. One of the more astonishing things to me is how they communicate both in quality and frequency. They make sure that the other one knows they are of utmost importance and respect to each other.

I'm Not A Mama's Boy I'm A Blessed Son

As I look at the efforts my Dad places in honoring my mother, I have always tried to in my more immature way do the same. This shows up in two different ways: to other women and to her. When it comes to other women, I have always tried to honor women generally but specifically the women that I've been romantically interested in have been the recipients of my efforts in the same vein that my father would. They've yet to be received in an open way and as I've always been "too much" or "annoying" but I see how these efforts in thoughtfulness and care light up my mom and I connect those efforts to how a man is supposed to be with his wife. It's all I can see. Her smiles and her radiance...all through the love.

Clearly, I have yet to enter my father's tax bracket and I do not have an Oedipus complex, but I love my mother dearly. I am very public with how much I care for her and have call her "My Number One Lady". To me she is a walking living and breathing proverbs 31 in the flesh. The fact that the passage says that her children will rise and call her blessed alone is evidenced in these words here. Society right now has an issue where a lot of males are so attached to their mothers that they are unable to ever actually grow up. Others are afraid of strong women and ironically the strength of their own mothers who already love them confuses them into shying away from strong women they could love in relationships because they feel that their masculinity is being challenged. The seek their mother in other women when they look for romantic relationships. Now for me my mother is tough as nails but as graceful as a cloud. She's as powerful as a hurricane but as sweet as a canary. She is balanced.

My mom has 5 kids and I truly believe that if something dire happening to any one of us she would become the female version of *Taken* and literally mow down, take out and remove whatever was in her way to get us to safety. She is why I have such high standards for women I'm interested in and high standards for myself. I believe that a man that is with my mother is man. A woman like her doesn't just fall out of the sky and isn't an accident she is a once in a lifetime. I see her work ethic, her grind, her intelligence and her vision. She can see things that aren't even fully understood to her. She passionately works to bring the utmost out of anyone. She's constantly pushing and pruning for greatness. In all of that she humbly just goes about the business of being herself. Even though she moves with an easy confidence of herself, she doesn't boast in her own accomplishments. Always quick to speak about those she's connected to, my mother will go on and on bragging about what one of her kids or her husband has done. The focus is almost never something she turns to herself. In the end she wants those she can influence to maximize their potential and she's never been one to just sit and speak to your potential she put effort behind making it happen. Even if the area that she's moving in and she may not be an expert she will get in and put in true effort towards success with a drive for excellence.

It's a real honor to be to be the son of Sheila Vaughn; I sometimes try and imagine what I saw the moment I was placed in her arms. I am the first child my mother had, and I imagine that when she first looked at me that everything that God has placed in a person of possible to love radiated from her. I wish I could remember what it was like to see her in those first few moments. She says I just looked at her and didn't even cry. I'd like to think it's because I was in complete safety. My whole life my mom has been a person I have always felt secure with being able to confide in. She knows so much about me as a person and how I think. I observe how she has treated people and my father and the family and that has bled into how I treat others and my family. She is incredibly passionate and is truly one of my favorite people that I know.

One of my favorite things about my mother ironically is one of her most frustrating attributes and that her ability and aim to push a frustrating situation towards a positive perspective. It can be the worst situation and my mother will try and see how to get some lesson, some piece of wisdom, something just anything that doesn't waste the situation. As I've grown into an adult looking to make my own decisions it would frustrate me that she's not allow me to stew in what's bothering me. I believe that many of us especially in society now want to invite people to pity parties when things aren't going our way. When someone won't take invitations to our pity parties, we tend to send them to someone who will come and join us. My mother was a person who would come to hear what's going on and then she'll shake up what's going on because the party is not going to stay the way it is if she's part of it. Her way of approaching a situation always is to listen and then point out where the silver lining is. Almost never do I want to hear it in fact because I'm so cerebral and she isn't, I'd fight her logically on it, but she would always remain steadfast in looking to where the situation could be used for growth.

I appreciate the quality of my mother to look for where a problem or frustration can be turned around into a win because it is instrumental in maximizing yourself in reaching your purpose. The people who allow themselves to remain stuck in where they are or the situation, they're experiencing never grow to a place of strength that would take them to another level. Imagine playing a video game and being stuck on a level you just can't get passed, no matter what you do. So, you go online and complain about how hard the level is and how the game isn't made to allow someone to get through the level. On all the forums you go to everyone is saying different things that are also along the lines of complaining about how hard the level is. What you don't know is that you must find a tool somewhere on the level that will allow you to pass to the next level but also will be pertinent to your success on the future levels to come. Without this tool you can't win the other levels at all. So, in all the noise of your complaining there's a voice that has been listening or reading your complaints. They don't know where the tool is, they don't even know you need one BUT what they do is start to suggest another perspective for your frustration. When you listen to this voice, you not only calm down you also see the level completely differently and no longer are looking to just get through it you see how you can THRIVE in it. Then you become a MASTER at the level and eventually become more than proficient and find the tool you need to succeed on the next level. What you don't notice is that now because you have put the work in to master the frustrating level with a new perspective you are now more than able and equipped to handle what's next. This experience is what it's like to be blessed to be encouraged by my mom. She sees potential in people and will come along side to not just hear your angst but then push you to see the situation in ways that you hadn't. Then when you view it differently you then move to a place where you not only succeed but you conquer.

In all this as big as her heart is and as much as she can cheer people towards their successes my mom will never seek to get any credit. She just sees opportunity to get things done and does it. She sees needs and works to fill them without making noise or drawing attention to what or why. She just has the mindset of "this isn't right, and it needs to be fixed" She starts looking for resources and throwing them into action. Sometimes my mom can leap before she looks and because neither me or my father are like that at times, we can have disagreements with her but she's all about filling needs. Her hands are almost never not on something that could be done.

I call her my number 1 Lady because I really have never come across a woman who does womanhood so well. She continues to adapt, grow and love with and effortless elegance that is sought after, prayed for, dreamt about and even studied. My mother is doing so much and so many things well that this whole book could be about her. When I wrote my first book, I had little mention of her influence in my life, but I had plenty about my father, and that was because of context but as she read it, she never even mentioned why she didn't have much words. She never searches for the spotlight she just does what she believes God has for her to do and that's the biggest impact she has ever had on my life. On that day when she first held me. If I knew God's voice then and could remember what he said to me just minutes old I'd like to believe he'd say something like "This woman will always love you, Caleb I picked her for you because she is a woman of integrity, class and wisdom. Caleb as you grow up, you'll need her love and grace. There is no need to cry because with her no matter where you are or what situation you may find yourself in, this woman will help get you through it. This is your mom, because I love you sweet child I give you to her" It was 3 days before I ever cried and that was because I had to let someone know I was hungry but I have to believe that I didn't cry at first because I knew my parents were people to keep me safe and secure even from the beginning.

Naturally as I've gotten older and marriage is a real possibility for my soon season my mom has made jokes about what will her role shift to and how will she be number 1 when my wife takes her place. I hadn't been able to come up with what to call her and one day I hope to know because my mom is immensely important to me. I call her once for sure every week and sometimes multiple times a week. I have an excellent relationship with her where she always can hear what's going on in my life. Even though I don't know what her "title" will be when I get married, I do know is that the way I look to treat my future wife will be somewhat of a tribute to her. Showing my mom that I love her because I treat a woman correctly just the way my mom expected me to interact with people. I also am attracted to women who are confident in themselves looking to solve problems. Those that are cheering other people on. I find those women attractive just as I've seen my mother sometimes verbally shout at the top of her lungs to push you on to victory. I look for those little things in women that I'd pursue subconsciously but still what I want in a wife and how I look to treat her flows from my relationship with Sheila Vaughn my number 1 Lady. I'm not a mama's boy but I am an intensely blessed son!

Everyone Else Is Taken

I'm a very cerebral person. I'm often in my head just pondering information and perspectives no topics. I'm working out the ways to see different points of view or solutions or I'm simply; ironically, just thinking. I believe my wandering mind's eye first was cultivated in grade school. My school was part of the Book It program that would reward students for reading a certain number of books and the reward was pizza hut pizza. If you ask my parents, I have always liked to eat, even then so reading to eat even more was a good motivation. In those early young reading days, I would gravitate to mysteries and sports books. Being that I enjoyed sports and being active so books on basketball, football and baseball were always favorites. In second grade was when I first started to watch basketball and football on TV. I also read Michael Jordan's autobiography in that season of my life. Naturally I was drawn to those stories and pictures painted through words. I would see myself in these games or watching the action almost as if I was in the crowd when the different events were happening. Reading on sports made me appreciate what could be learned from them even more. The lessons and celebrations all were given a new perspective when reading what different moments; whether fiction or non-fiction, would mean to a person through sports. So much of what I would look to apply to my life I have learned through sports, but a lot of my initial approach was from understanding the perspectives and lessons from the words of other people.

Mysteries came into my life later in about 4th grade my God-mother gave me a box set of The Hardy Boys books. She gifted me the first original 10 books and I ate them up. I absolutely devoured the material and the stories. To follow two boys as they'd grow into men solving different puzzles and challenges. They had different relationships grow and have different peaks and valleys, but the central focus was that these two brothers could solve mysteries. The best detectives in mysteries always must take in the facts they are given and put together pieces that aren't readily there. They must look to place themselves in perspectives that aren't naturally their own as they try to live a piece of a story through someone else's experiences. Reading these types of books really allowed me to create images and see visions of things from others perspective with only some facts. One simple way to explain it is like seeing a movie being put together in my mind. As I get different facts about a situation, I'm almost watching the story play out on the screen behind my eyes just as vividly as if I were to have seen it in a theater.

As I've gotten older this process has caused me to consider numerous topics and experiences from different vantage points than I would naturally. The process in my mind has sped up as well and as I continue to get to know myself better it also becomes easier to articulate to others what I'm seeing and understanding. Believe me it's frustrating to get stuck at a fork in the road in your mind and need just a piece of information to go down either path that you're contemplating but you're not sure which one is correct. So, you're trying to lead someone else down all the trails you went to get to the fork in the road, but the solution would've been so clear if they could just provide you that one piece...Frustrating!

All of this has led me to create a way of processing that is all my own. I fully know that as I take in information that I'm working through it all to be sure I stand by my own conclusions and communicate to others through maybe why they should consider mines as well. So often people aren't spending the time understanding themselves. They haven't sought their purpose or even what is important to them they don't know how they think or believe. They just have grown to follow everyone else's way of thinking. When you want to walk into your future with excellence and maximize yourself you must consider how YOU think. What is important to YOU!

History has an ironic way of showing how something can be applied even if the items it's being applied to are different or even opposing. Using two very recognizable figures in history; Martin Luther King and Adolf Hitler. Both men were influential leaders whose decisions changed the course of history for millions. Both stood for two enormously different things and success for one was remarkably different looking than the other. However, as different as their motives and goals were one thing that they shared is that they were totally convinced that they were correct in what they were fighting for. They had the self-confidence and inner belief in themselves AND what their goals were that they sought to convince others to follow them. They were not followers waiting on a confirmation they were people of action pressing towards a goal.

Too often people spend lots of time on social media wallowing in the realm of hashtags and retweets looking to find reasons for their worth to be validated. These people are not thinking for themselves they're thinking for approval. People will continue to circulate the same ideas without ever posing solutions because so many other people think like them. At the end of the day no new perspectives are ever injected and no leader steps up to bring any resolutions. It is important to understand how you think so that you can think for yourself. If you have a set of values and understandings when you come across ideas that conflict with yours then you then are presented with an opportunity to grow and bring something new to your perspective or you can sharpen the idea that has been brought to you with your perspective. That all starts with knowing you and how you think. What is important to you and why. Learning how you communicate through your thoughts and owning what you think in turn builds the self-assurance that what you believe is what you believe. To do this effectively you have to be able to consider perspectives outside of yourself and synthesize them so that you arrive at conclusions that can be used in a valuable way.

When I was in grade school, I spent so much time being physically alone that I've always gotten to just imagine and see the perspectives and stories of others through what I read. Books are so much freer than movies because in movies even though there's possibly a fictional story being told there's still not a lot of room to imagine outside of what is shown on the screen. Even if you do imagine something the value of that thought is generally confirmed or denied of that worth by the end of the movie. In books the addition of the thoughts of the characters brings a different dimension to a story. Now as a reader you have motive and then you can see action. As I spent all that time spending time seeing motives and actions, I would consider perspectives and think of the why's behind the actions. I apply that as an adult, when hearing someone's story and their thought process I'm able to see myself walking in their shoes almost like my eyes have been traded for theirs as I begin to work to understand their beliefs and perspectives. As I bring motives and ideas together now, I can effectively communicate with them and have fruitful dialogue ahead.

Exceed And Defeat The Expectations

Caleb- Hebrew translation: Bold and Faithful like a dog. When I was a kid, I was first told that my name meant to be bold. From this understanding as far back as I can remember I have always declared that I'm not afraid of anything. Sure, I've been nervous of potential outcomes of situations or have felt uneasy about different potential experiences, but I honestly can say I haven't been afraid of an outcome. Being bold and courageous is in me. It's part of who I am. I think that's part of the reason I've been able to live without fear is the fact that I've never been one that has been widely appreciated or liked. Since I haven't been appreciated by many, I don't know what it's like to disappoint many people. In fact, the people who I'm most pained about disappointing is my family and myself. More times than not those people are cheering me on in pursuits of my goals.

I've always seen fear as an annoyance. It always steals from potential, joy and bliss. Don't misinterpret what I'm saying that there aren't scary things or that danger isn't real but an acronym for fear that my mother told me when I was young was False Evidence Appearing Real. That's exactly what fear is. It's a misplacement of perspective and using that perspective to change the trajectory of one's actions. If you use a perspective of how something may fail or seeing all the pain in potential, then you'll never see an opportunity for that thing to thrive. If you change the perspective and use a lens that looks to see that things blossom and hopes for its success awe inspiring revelations and experiences are to then happen.

One thing I've heard about is how a lot of people don't want to bring children into the world because of how crazy they think it's getting. It's always disheartening to hear because these stories always come from people who want children, but they are afraid that it would be selfish of them to bring a person into a place that seems so terrible. On the surface their holding back is noble, but the reality is that their decision is motivated by fear. One of the main aims of fear is to hold you back from ever doing all that you are supposed to. What better way to impact others and the world is there than to have children that you can equip to engage with the world properly? What happens if all the well-meaning and seemingly noble positive parents decided to sit out of parenting due to fear? Chaos would be allowed to grow and fester as the stance in oppositions of truth and peace would grow weaker. The true change and elevation in society will come through a people who are willing to stand up in boldness pushing for what is right as they inject that courageousness into an auspicious legacy. A legacy that will infiltrate and infect culture, to ultimately affect elevation of purpose, and leave a lasting effective impact on lives.

If you make decisions from a perspective in which fear is the motive, you'll make unwise and likely inefficient decisions. As from the acronym the evidence you're using isn't accurate, it isn't real. A person who has vision challenges and uses glasses to see clearly need the proper prescription in order to see correctly. If the prescription of the lens that they're looking through is incorrect then they won't be able to properly discern the world around them. In turn causing them to inefficiently and possibly dangerously participate in the world around them. They may be slower to move because they aren't sure as to how to truly exist in the world. All their decisions of movement would be something they'd question where they may possibly not move at all. However, when they put on the correct prescription and can see through a lens that provides the right perspective and they can move in boldness and confidence into what they are looking to do. That is the same way it goes for operating in fear or boldness. We must seek the correct perspective and evidence rather than allowing counterfeit information to cloud our judgement and hinder our progression. The truth gives confidence and it's available to access; the lies just are a bit easier to see. You might have to put effort into moving the falsehoods out of the way and step forward to beat fear and be able to operate in boldness.

Living a life steeped in fear will bind you from seeing all who you could be. You will always struggle to get to where you are purposed to be if you never step out into things that you have never done. A wise quote from an unknown speaker says, "The comfort zone is a beautiful place, but nothing ever grows there." If you never take the opportunity to see what you can do because you're so comfortable where you are you won't get all that's to be for you. There are people who live complete lives of stagnation mediocrity because they were never willing to step out and see what was outside of their comfort zone. A lot of people get so locked into what they are seeing and experiencing in their comfort that they don't even see life passing them by. There are people whose lives depend on you. You have a reason for being and for the time that in which you exist. If you stay trapped in concern for what could be simply because it's unknown your life will never truly be fulfilled and the lives you are to reach as well as the legacy, you are to leave will never be realized.

Best Effort No Matter The Audience

When interviewing for jobs I often was asked about what I consider my greatest strengths and how do I leverage that in the workplace. Now, because I liked to be remembered and I wanted to give a real answer I would avoid things like "I'm a hard worker" or "Team player" I figured those were things many of those that I was competing with would also say so I would think about what about me is something that I bring to work that others really don't; I came to realize looking in my personal life and work life my greatest strength is my integrity. Many people consider themselves leaders and if they don't see themselves as leaders currently, they hope to be in positions of influence one at some point. Organizations are always better off if they are led by people of integrity so much more are the people who lead their lives with integrity. I have always been a man who follows through with his word and seeks to be dependable. I look to be a person that doesn't give a leader, who is delegating tasks reason to be concerned. They don't have to wonder if I'm going to complete the task and if I'd do it will it be correctly done. Most challenges in my career have a solution rooted in a sense of integrity. I mentioned that a solid leader would evaluate where they are as they look to progress forward. In order to be able to move forward they would need information, obtained in earnest and integrity.

When building structures such as homes or large skyscrapers often there's a discussion into the time put into focusing on the making sure the foundation is strong. Many times, the phrase structural integrity is thrown around as it's understood that without a solid foundation everything that will come afterwards that goes on top of the foundation will fail if there's a weak foundation. A lot of times we don't focus on creating solid foundations in our lives and things collapse on us. Making creating a strong foundation isn't always fun and oftentimes can be quite tedious. Even in the mundane and sometimes even frustrating moments, it's THOSE moments that is when the foundation's integrity is most refined. Those are the most important parts in the building process because it's instrumental in allowing any possible valuable progression.

When I played sports in school, I would receive very challenging feedback at times from coaches. Even though it would be hard to take challenging feedback at times I still would learn and grow through those times. I often didn't appreciate the way the feedback was delivered but the message was something that I would take in because I wanted to succeed so badly. I wanted to have a strong foundation grounded in the fundamentals because I believed that the consequences of failing at being sure on the details were usually quick and blatant. If I hadn't worked to improve areas of my game and focused on the details, I could possibly come across an opponent who could expose those same areas. When you're immediately exposed and defeated because you didn't do the work on the little things then you understand their importance very clearly. In our lives sometimes these types of stark failures aren't as blatant. However, usually when there is a failure it ends up being a major problem. It's something that might have been brewing for multiple years and ends up being a breakdown that damages the lives of many others, especially when that failure is when a person is leadership or has people looking up to them. Those meltdowns almost always come back to doing a lot of little things wrong. When a person exhibits true integrity, things don't even get to the point of major failure because they handle the small things as they come because they are building for a future and vision.

My focus in harnessing my integrity is doing the small things right and maximizing where I'm at so that I have a solid foundation for my future leadership; that's my focus now. I follow through on my word and do everything I can to do what I can with excellence. In order to be the greatest success, I can I make sure to do well with what I have currently before I could be entrusted with anymore. Strong effective leaders must display integrity to properly encourage those they lead towards the vision for the organization.

A lot of times we see our peers or figures that we respect do amazing things, we see them operate in spaces that we wish to be in ourselves but it's easy to focus on when what's being done looks easy when the reality is that the road to get to a point in which it would look easy was actually a hard one to travel. It requires patience and diligence to harness what is required in order to reach the highest levels of excellence. The refining of the details is built in obscurity. No one just arrives on the scene ready and made. There are trials, there's angst and times where quitting seems like the best option. However, when tapping out seems like a way to ease the pain of the struggle. That's when you must remember to check the pulse of your purpose and it will continue to beat if you are alive. If you are still breathing, you have a purpose. If you are still here you have purpose and it is, your charge to not let that purpose die inside of you. Just because it's hard. It might seem like too much. BUT you were not made of mediocrity and not formed for futility. Stay committed to the process even in the background where you may not be seen. Once you make it to the stage, because of the fires that you have been forged in the pressure will not destroy you.

When you are pushing forward in purpose you may not fully grasp why you can't quit but it's because invariably there are people whose purpose depends on you fulfilling yours. There are legacies that are to be birthed out of your commitment and there's change that you must champion. Without you looking to bring the reason you are placed in the world at this time to fulfillment, someone else may miss out on the very key to unlock the door to their destiny. You may be exactly what someone needs to accomplish remarkable things in their life. Don't give up. Don't give in. Find the passion, hold on to it and keep the desire and drive; lit in your chest.

<u>Set Your Time By Me</u>

A lot of people wonder why they can't move forward in their lives. Some feel stagnant in relationships and others are challenged in their workplaces. There are people who have a desire to see their current reality change and they don't know what can be done to get where they're looking to get to. They have this amazing idea of what they can see for their life but what they experience daily isn't what they get experience. I believe one of the biggest areas that hinder many of us in getting to these next levels in life is our faithfulness in honoring where we currently are. It's easy to be excited about what you want to do or even where you see yourself in the future, but can you maintain what you currently have? How you steward what you currently have speaks towards how you'd maintain a future blessing or elevation later.

I believe a great example of where this unearned promotion where one is elevated before they are prepared is in winning the lottery. Much is documented about lottery winners and how after they've won astronomical jackpots that their lives are ruined following their big win. Oftentimes these people are those that were previously living from paycheck to paycheck. They didn't have much, if any savings or they simply had no plan. So, when they're suddenly given more money than they had ever expected to see in their life they aren't able to make a transition into a new lifestyle because they hadn't been preparing for it. They haven't built up the skills to tend to their new fortune well. Imagine getting the ability to do everything that you desired to ever do but when you get it the things you already have and cherished dissolve. Lottery winners have gotten into many different types of unhealthy living decisions because they had a new access to things they hadn't before. Whether it be harsh drugs and alcohol or connecting with dangerous people. Some people actual blow their money continuing to gamble because they're not satisfied in their winnings they just want to continue to try and live where they pursue more. They're not satisfied.

Not everyone can relate to a lottery winner or coming into a new fortune but many of us would like to grow beyond where we are or at least maximize what we're currently doing. One thing about me is that I'm always looking to maximize what I can do and sometimes frustrate myself that I'm not where I want to be. I'm incredibly competitive and visionary, so oftentimes when what I'm seeing for my future and where I'm currently at aren't lining up I can get lost in where my focus is. As I've grown, I've seen share of opportunities to get all I can out of where I was even though it wasn't where I wanted to stay. There's a delicate balance in being a driven person. On one hand it's an excellent quality to have where you're looking to grow, learn and improve any and every way you think to do so. However, on the other hand you can't be so driven that you are unable to grow where you are and even take in the lessons of your current space. Also, if you get caught up in comparison of where you are in relation to others who may seem further along you also run the risk of never being truly maximizing your potential.

The summer of 2016 was one of the most challenging experiences of my life. I had left my first job that I accepted out of college after only being in the role for 6 months. The situation I came out of was one that I could not remain in and be healthy. However, when I resigned, I left before I had another job lined up. This set up for an incredibly trying 9-month journey from January to August of that year for me. I had already begun prospecting for jobs in the couple weeks before my actual resignation, so I believed that I'd probably be only out of a job for a short while, while living off my savings for a couple months. Through 2 months of looking and my savings running out I had to go on unemployment assistance and to aid in maintaining my bills. I also would eventually have to expand my job focus from just career jobs in my field to including part time jobs so that I could still pay to live. This led me to the most humbling summer of my working life. I was college educated, with multiple notches of experience on my resume. I graduated a semester late, so I had more time before launching into the world. I had made many connections leading up to my graduation but still I found myself in a survival situation with a lease that had to be paid and needing to eat so to make ends meet I found myself first working at a Kwik Fill gas station and then at a KFC.

I lived right down the street from both stores and it really was simple for me to pursue openings in them. With Kwik Fill I had already worked at a location near my parents' house when I was looking for work post grad so I figured it would be easy to get back in to a position there as I would continue to look for work. I calculated the hours I would need to work to pay my rent and if I maintained that I'd have some free time to be able to use in looking for another job. So, the plan was in place and I was hired on the spot when I was called in for the interview and started 2 days later. Once I started, I was back to the duties of stocking shelves and working a cash register. I was counting cigarettes and issuing out lottery tickets. I had to clean the store and check the gas levels. I was doing all my job duties earning New York state minimum wage. I worked at this job consistently each week for 3 months. Since this was a 24-hour store with a set block for hours, I worked hours I did not like. Sometimes I worked at times I did not want to be working but I had to. The one single reason I left was that I wasn't getting the hours that I was promised when I first started.

Unlike the job I left after college I was able to earn my position with KFC before leaving Kwik Fill. The manager was incredibly friendly as was the whole staff. It was a blessing that the manager decided to pay me as much as a supervisor even though I had no experience in the company. His sole reason was because I already had a bachelor's degree. In many ways this job was even more humbling than the gas station starting from day 1 I was a cashier and was being trained by a 16-year-old. I vividly remember the year she was born! In fact, most of my co-workers there were 21 and younger and no one; including the manager and assistant managers had college degrees. Even though I didn't like what I was doing in the sense of what I went to school for and was looking to earn I was grateful that I had income that would allow me to at least live as I figured it out. I no longer had to worry about having enough to pay my bills with the hours and wage I had. My concern now was still to continue to apply to career jobs and be a strong team member at KFC. I was consistent in never being late to a shift and being attentive to our customers. I reached a point where some customers would mention to my manager on days, I had off that they wished I was there to take their order.

I was always just doing the best I could. I figure that since I was there, I might as well do my job the best I could with the best attitude I could have. It's easy to be stuck in frustration with your situation when it doesn't look like how you imagined it or want it to be like and have that steal your focus when greater or simply a blessing might be on the other side of a positive attitude. A very wise man shared with me a message that an incredible woman shared with him years ago that can apply to so many things in life. "Your attitude is the difference." It's just 5 words but there's so much that you can do with this sentiment. Your attitude can literally dynamically shift so much about your life depending on how you let it.

Both directions for an attitude whether positive or negative always looks for opportunity. Negative attitudes look for the chances to be drab and downtrodden, never seeing a solution to succeed or shift the situation. Oftentimes negative attitudes drag and shackle the one carrying it as well as those they affect. A positive attitude looks for solutions, see the opportunities for success and completion. The wearer of a positive attitude tends to energize and uplift those around them and that they engage with.

As I carried a positive attitude in to my job at KFC daily in engaging with customers and my team members I was given an opportunity to see the power in a positive attitude. An older gentleman came in and ordered his food at a lull of a time in the day.

We made his order and were running breaks. I was helping in the back and generally busy. I remember he came up after it seemed he had finished and asked for some butter and honey for his biscuit. I came up seeing he needed help saying, "Hey how can I help?" and he told me of his need, and I changed my gloves and quickly got them. I could see where he sat, and it seemed as if his food was done but nonetheless, I got his honey and butter and asked if he is needing anything more then I went to my work again. 5 minutes or so later he came back up. At this point I'm concerned because customers only come back more times when something is wrong. He specifically asked for me to the counter so I'm just KNOWING I did something wrong. Anyways I say, "hello sir is everything ok, did we get everything for you?" Now the next thing he said to me I can remember everything about it. I can even see the colors in the room. It was as if it was just him and I in that moment, it was something completely unbelievable. He said "I'm retired, and my wife has passed. So, every day I wake up and go to the bank and get extra money and ask the Lord; Father tell me who I'm to bless today." "When you came up to help me with such a warm attitude God told me "that's him". So, the man slid $50 dollars in my hand plus his change that would've been for his meal. Then walked out.

In my life I've heard of God working through people for others in challenging times. I've even watched a movie or two where someone just couldn't catch a break somehow would get one. Sure the $50 didn't maybe pay all my rent or anything but it was a sure sign that I was not at all forgotten. I don't even recall what I said to the man. I don't even remember seeing him walk out. I just remember going to the back and crying. I was so frustrated and felt so low. I felt like a failure. I had let myself and my family down. I was a disappointment. How was it that I was working at KFC? Why am I in a situation receiving state assistance to pay my rent AND am on a payment plan with my apartment complex? Somehow someway I was on God's mind enough that he'd have an old man come and eat some chicken when I was working and need some butter and honey. I would get reminded that as I would remain consistent and keep a positive attitude my situation would change, and he would not and has not forgotten about me.

Even I as I recant this story and almost every time, I think about it I cry some. It's at the worst moments in life where the smallest break is all you need to understand that you're still seen and still matter. Even when you don't feel it, someone is on assignment to change and affect our world. Someone is sent to assist you though your situation. Even when it's most frustrating keep a positive attitude and strive on. Things will change.

A few weeks after that experience I was given a call from Travelers Insurance. This was in July of 2016. They wanted to interview me, I didn't even recall ever applying but I investigated the job they said I applied for and liked the description, so I agreed to an interview. In the interview I was sitting down with 2 executives and a senior manager of the local office. I was told at the conclusion of my interview that there was another position to also post for, for consideration. I did so just for the insurance (no pun intended) and was given the job. This job was one I didn't interview for at all. The next call I got was about pay and start dates. The manager I ended up reporting to was given my paperwork the weekend before my first day as she wasn't even part of my hiring process. This new position paid me more than the one I first left in January, I would have more vacation time, a more expansive retirement package and more flexible work with a lot more support. At the end of the day this job was a lot better than the one I left to start the terrible 2016 summer. Through that summer I remained consistent where I worked. All my responsibilities were priorities that I completed regularly. I was reliable and maintained a positive attitude. I learned so much about who I am under pressure. I learned how to value all people in a way I hadn't considered. I also learned humility that I wouldn't have experienced in any other way. Most importantly I learned that in staying committed to the mission, as you push toward your goal doesn't mean that you won't face frustration. In the end, if you keep trying, and maintain the faith that the season of frustration will eventually end, you will be better than where you began.

Fuel Up

Your purpose is not for you. I am a shy person and only feel comfortable in long discourse with people I know and feel comfortable with. However, I will step out and speak as my purpose is to help other's reach theirs. I love to encourage and cheer people on as they reach their goals and see their dreams become reality. Even though I'm not always sure what the best words or way to go about my expression I look to remain locked in to conversations as they happen. I want to know the stories of people and I value them as the passion they carry with them is sacred. My daily place where I stand and offer encouragement is my social media. I used to be such a complainer and victim with a lot of my expression. My mindset shift to victory and encouragement has led me to craft different anecdotes and small quotes. These pieces of thought have blessed me first on my push in purpose to I want to give you some fuel as you face to your future. I don't want to give any analysis of these quotes because I want them to speak to you and for you to get what you're supposed to out of them.

"Life isn't about perfection it's about progression"

"Don't let yourself be defined by something worth less than you"

"The world needs a maturing version of you, not a cheap version of someone you admire"

"When you combine your gift with your calling you become unstoppable"

"When trying to achieve something, the difficulty isn't the problem, it's the discipline"

"Comparison will consistently cloud the clarity of the call on your life"

"If you are invisible to others it's only because their vision is limited, not your value"

"Are your decisions limited by your resources or are your resources limited by your decisions"

"If what you stand for doesn't bother anybody then it probably won't impact anybody"

"The revelation of your future does not come from within you"

"You can't find the fullness of your purpose until you're willing to let go of control"

"Don't let the perception of other someone else's actions change your actions and how you live your life"

"You will never bare fruit if you keep listening to people that tell you what you want to hear"

"When you can afford to quit; you can't quit"

"Don't serve your talents, use your talents to serve"

"Sometimes the best way to measure distance isn't to look back and see how far you've gone, but to look ahead and see how close you are"

"Being ordinary is easy…excellence never is"

Face To The Future

It's never too late to start living and until you're gone you always must run in the lane of your purpose. There is a specific reason and assignment that you are in the space and time that you are reading these words. There are people that depend on your fulfilling the assignment of your life. Don't look to other lanes and focus on the path that you're walking; there's less traffic there! It's easy to hear about the amazing things that people do in their lives and seem to have come from pain or overcome a lot to get there. It's easy to see the giants of history and maybe want to be like them but feel unqualified. If there's nothing the words in this book sticks with you, this is the message that I want you to take. I want you to understand that in all that you have experienced, all the amazing bliss and beautiful experiences. As you consider all the frustration, feelings of failure and seemingly never-ending pain. Consider how you're able to weld the power of your strengths and face the concern in your present weaknesses. When your weakness speaks don't listen to what your weakness says. It's all in YOU and YOU are enough. Everything that you need has been placed inside of you for success. So, walk into your future with unshakable confidence. All you have is all you need.